CHEERLEADER FAITH

CHEERLEADER FAITH

Team Spirit for the Cancer Patient
What To Do When Trouble Comes!

Marge Houchins

Library of Congress Control Number: 2011911391
ISBN: Hardcover   978-1-4628-4566-8
                 Softcover   978-1-4628-4565-1
                 Ebook   978-1-4628-4567-5

Unless otherwise noted, all Scripture quotations used in this book are taken from the
New American Standard Translation of the Bible.

Faith Alive Ministry
408 N. Logan
Olathe, Ks. 66061

e-mail faith_word1@yahoo.com

For a complete list of materials please write or email for a catalog to the above
address.

This book was printed in the United States of America.

To order additional copies of this book, contact:
Xlibris Corporation
1-888-795-4274
www.Xlibris.com
Orders@Xlibris.com
102011

CONTENTS

Dedication 7

Introduction 9

Chapter 1   A Little History... 11

Chapter 2   The Support System.....................................21

Chapter 3   The Treatment Begins 24

Chapter 4   Faith Tested 30

Chapter 5   Marge's Journal..38

Chapter 6   Captain of the Team Departs 45

Prayer for Healing 50

Prayer for Salvation and Baptism in the Holy Spirit 51

References 53

Photo Gallery..57

Rarely does a person experience the richness of life that is so full of all your dreams . . . my husband was a champion in my eyes. A man full of the love of God, wisdom beyond his years . . . . always aiming to please me but keep his integrity with his Lord.

I dedicate this book to Pastor Jerry Houchins with my deepest love and respect and gratitude for twenty-four beautiful years full of wonderful memories. His strength and courage will ever and always be etched on the pages of my mind.

INTRODUCTION

I went to a Ladies Retreat and the theme was What Kind of Legacy Will You Leave?" What will your family and friends say about you after you depart this earth? That gave me cause to ponder. My grand children tell me if it wasn't for me and Jerry, their family might not be in church serving the Lord today.

You see, before Jerry got sick, they were not in church. They watched how strong he was during those six years that he fought the good fight of faith against cancer. They watched him stay strong in the faith, even at times when it didn't look like he would make it another day. They watched him love His Lord, each time he got a negative report. They watched him not blame God for what he was experiencing, but stayed true to his faith. They were able to see the miracle God gave him during remission.

Our grandchildren watched us maintain a positive faith. They watched me cheer Jerry on during the battle of his life. They watched me be a support system to him whenever he needed me to be. They watched the strength of my faith in the Lord rise to the top when Jerry went home to be with the Lord. The reason I could stand in the midst of sadness because I was assured of the word of God that says, *"Precious in the sight of the Lord is the death of his saints."*

They watched us know what to do 'when trouble comes.' Not only did they see me and Jerry fight the good fight of faith during his years of dealing with cancer, but they also watched how we reacted when our thirty-three year old daughter was killed in an automobile accident.

The legacy was in place, and we believe the Lord will see to it that it will continue for many generations to come.

One night before we became Pastors, Jerry had a dream that he saw his deceased father. He was young and robust with new bib overalls on and he was coming out of a corn field holding some ears of corn. Jerry ran to him, then he woke up. He was troubled about the dream's meaning.

I had been asking God to use me in more prophetic gifts. About a week after Jerry had his dream, I felt like I fell into a trance, and I saw Jerry's father coming out of the corn field towards him. Jerry ran and fell at his feet. He said, "No, son, get up. You have to go and gather the harvest," and handed him thirteen years of fresh corn.

At that time, there were thirteen members in the church where his dad had been the Pastor. This was a confirmation we were to Pastor the church. Of course, there were a couple that left during the interim period of waiting for a new Pastor to come. When we began to Pastor the Lighthouse Church, one family left the church, and then there were eight remaining. In Bible numerology, eight means a new beginning.

It was certainly a new beginning for us. We lived our dream as active Pastors in Beardstown, Illinois for the next eight years. We were blessed God used us to build the church up to ninety-four at one time. We were thrilled doing what we knew God had called us to do.

Due to the battle we ended up involved in, we had to walk away from our home, our community, and our church we dearly loved, but we're thankful our family was able to watch as we humbly threw ourselves on God. We could have become bitter and angry at God, but we chose not to. I give God all the praise and thanks for what He's done in my life, and in my family's life. I'm thankful for the legacy me and Jerry were able to leave behind to our children, grand children, and generations to come.

I also give God all the glory for giving me and Jerry wisdom to know what to do when trouble comes. Yes, I truly enjoyed my role as a Pastor's wife, but I was thankful God called me to be a cheerleader and support system during the final days of my husband's life. I would not have wanted to do anything else when the trouble came.

CHAPTER ONE

A Little History

Imagine standing before a crowd of people saying, "I Do," to the very familiar marriage vow, "Do you take this man for better or worse, for richer or poorer, in sickness and in health,"

I never dreaming that some day you might have to face the negative side to that vow. We did.

Our wedding day, January 4, 1985, was one of the happiest days of my life. Just like other wedding days before and after ours, I was focused on the day at hand, excited about marrying the man I loved. As my father-in-law performed our wedding ceremony, I happily repeated my marriage vows, and not once did the thought cross my mind that in the near future I would become my husband's cheer leader and support system while we journeyed through a six-year battle of lymphoma cancer and GI bleed. We would walk through the valley of the shadow of death, and God would be with us every step of the way.

The saying, 'You don't have a clue,' certainly applied in our case.

We spoke our wedding vows that wintry day in January, over twenty-five years ago, having no idea what was ahead. Our hearts burned with love for one another, trusting we would experience only the good version of our marriage vows. Even if we would have known what lie ahead, we wouldn't have changed a thing. I definitely would have still been there for him.

After my husband passed away, my sister asked me, "Marge, how did you survive all you went through, caring for Jerry as he fought that dreaded disease?" Her question caused me to ponder, and motivated me to write this book.

I had never thought of myself as a cheerleader. When I was in school, I was in the pep squad, and was a majorette in the marching bad, but never a cheerleader; however, I became one for Jerry whenever he needed me to.

Jerry was a very active person, hardly ever idle, and enjoyed doing for others when we met and got married. He was healthy, hardly ever sick except for spinal meningitis he contracted when he was in the second grade, and he never forgot that God instantly healed him! He was a hard worker and great provider for our family. He preached the word with power and left a tremendous influence on many lives. A great example of that power was when his sister passed away during a church service one Sunday morning.

The service had just begun people were worshipping when Jerry's niece came to the platform and tugged on his sleeve and said, "Uncle Jerry, something is wrong with Grandma. He quickly left the platform and went to her seat. Her eyes had rolled back in her head and she did not have a pulse. Of course everything stopped.

Jerry laid hands on her head and shouted, "Devil, not here and not now." I take authority over death now in the name of Jesus.

Wilma, I speak to your spirit to come back into your body now in the NAME OF JESUS. She drew a deep breath with a gasp for air and her spirit was obedient to the prayer of faith. She had heart problems and had a pace-maker. The para—medics arrived and took her to the hospital and they confirmed she had indeed died.

She lived several months after this and had another attack while in the hospital and passed away. She had those months to spend time with her family and prepare for her departure for heaven.

She was a wonderful Christian lady. She was so dedicated to the helps ministry. You could count on her to keep the kitchen organized. She prepared many meals for God's people. She made a decision to depart, she was tired of the fight to stay healthy.

Jerry did not have a College education, so at times his speech often ungrammatical. However, he loved God with everything he had, he was steadfastly committed to God and to His Word, and he didn't rest until he saw God move in the lives of those that needed Him.

He had so much compassion for people and the ministry. He prayed for at least an hour every day, it didn't matter what the schedule for the day was, he made sure he spent time with the Lord to start the day. For enjoyment, we raised Missouri Fox Trotter horses together, and were thrilled to win the World Grand Championship Model Stallion in 1999, in Ava, Missouri.

We later moved to Beardstown, Illinois. My husband was self-employed, owning his own heating, air—conditioning and electrical company. Some years later, God called him to pastor the Lighthouse Church in Beardstown.

Jerry said yes to the ministry, and being the type of person who sold out to whatever he chose to do, he walked away from raising horses, and sold his business. The new owners who purchased the business got into some financial trouble, and knowing he wanted to serve God one hundred percent, and being the good-hearted man he was, he forgave their debt.

He loved serving God with his whole being. He was able to teach and preach from life's experiences, and of course, he had a great testimony of God miraculously healing him of the spinal meningitis in his early years. You don't forget those God times.

Time marched on, and he began having physical symptoms, and he had no doubts God would heal him, but an instantaneous healing wasn't to come this time.

Jerry's symptoms worsened so he made the decision to go see the doctor. Of course, she asked why he waited so long before coming for treatment. From his point of view, why not wait? He'd experienced God's healing first-hand, and we were accustomed to believing God, even when we had to wait on answers to prayer.

God is always faithful, so the reason for not going to see the doctor was an easy one for him—*he wanted to stand in faith for his healing.*

Yes, we knew God gave wisdom to doctors, we knew God's healing is not always instant, we knew He sends healing in many ways, and we knew it does not always come the way we prefer.

While his symptoms continued to progressively worsen, naturally, we had been praying. Where was the same God who had healed him of spinal meningitis? We had stood and prayed, stood and prayed, but we knew we were in desperate need of God's wisdom.

Jerry was struggling to breathe, he could not lay down, and had to sit up all night to be able to catch his breath. He had many sleepless nights.

Large lumps had formed on the back of his head and side of his neck, he had lost twenty pounds, and is energy level had dropped drastically.

Although he was diligent about his words, his prayers, his trust in God for healing, he must have known he had to see our local doctor. He went for a visit. When he came home, he said what no person ever wants to hear, "Doctor Wyatt thinks I have cancer and need to see a specialist."

When he told me what the doctor had said, we both were very cautious about our words. Being cautious wasn't new for us, but we were even more vigilant. Why so cautious about our words?

We knew the words spoken from our mouths would set our course.

Emotions are raging during the very worst time of our lives, and trust me, it is not easy to guard your lips!

Proverbs 18:21 Death and life are in the power of the tongue; and those who love it will eat its fruit.

Doctor Wyatt set up an appointment to see a pulmonary specialist, and in 2003, Jerry was diagnosed with fourth stage non-Hodgkin's B-Cell lymphoma cancer. The disease had progressed throughout his body. The majority of his lymph nodes were affected. He had a large cancerous mass in his stomach. His lungs showed Mestastic cancer. The specialist advised we begin C H O P, which is the acronym for a chemotherapy regimen used in the treatment of non—Hodgkin lymphoma. In scientific terms, C H O P stands for Clophosphamide, Hdroxydaunorubicin

(Doxorubicin), Oncovin (Vincristine), and prednisone/prednisolone.

In my terms, the acronym C H O P is hardly palatable.

Jerry was a man of faith, a minister, Pastor of the Lighthouse Church in Beardstown, Illinois for over seven years. He knew God's healing power, he'd seen many people healed over his lifetime, he'd seen many answers to prayers over the years. What happened?

Why did we have to face this trial? Yes, we. In any true marriage, even though one spouse is directly affected, any loving spouse is indirectly affected at a minimum. Why did we have to hear the word cancer? Why did we have to hear the words C H O P ?

What now? Our faith is now being put being put to the test. Do we throw it all out the window? Do we begin screaming, "NO!

NO! NO!" Do we throw a temper tantrum, get mad, and blame God like so many others when something horrible happens? Do we throw a pity party? Do we act arrogantly and think to ourselves, 'I'm serving You, and this is how You treat me?'

People of faith should not 'react' to bad news in a negative reaction.

And if we do, we have a problem and need to straighten out our thinking because our thinking produces a negative attitude. Negative thinking and a negative attitude are enemies of faith. Remember, the world was framed by the 'words of God!' God spoke right because we thought right. We're made in God's image, so our words are powerful. If we think wrong, then wrong words will stream out of our mouth. *"Out of the heart the mouth speaks"* the Bible says.

God has given us His word, which is heart and mind; His wisdom.

What are we going to do with His heart and mind that He's openly revealed to us in the written word of God—the Bible? *He's magnified His word above His name!* The word of God is an unstoppable force, *sharper than any two-edged sword,* given to every son and daughter of God! For God's word to properly and fully work in a child of God's life, we have to know what it says.

Do we realize how important His word is?

We had to depend on God's word like we never had when we were thrown into a battle we didn't want to find ourselves in. C H O P had started. During this time of aggressive medical intervention, we saw many of God's wonders. Jerry never experienced any type of nausea, sickness or weakness in his body. After chemo treatments, we would leave the hospital and go out to eat dinner. He would continue doing normal tasks like cleaning the car or whatever else was needed. I was still working a job at the time, so he would even clean the house for me every Friday.

He continued to preach from the pulpit, only missing two Sundays while we were in the hospital waiting for his diagnosis.

I don't want to appear that I'm minimizing what he went through it was no picnic by any means. We had to stand on the Word of God to pull us through this. We read lots of books from people that had overcome cancer. Dodie Osteen's book, 'Healed of Cancer,' was an inspiration to both of us. One day she called Jerry on the phone while he was in the hospital just to encourage him to keep fighting. Her kindness meant the world to both of us. She was a cheerleader on our team and didn't realize it!

To be a true support system for anyone, you must be able to be live in victory in your own personal life, and if you're able to do that, you know your true source is God. You know your victories are from believing God, and what God says.

At some point in your walk with God, your faith will be challenged.

What will you do? What would you do if a doctor told you that you, your spouse or a child has cancer? When a hard trial comes, what will you do in the heat of the battle? Will you give up? Will you stand? Will you become fearful? Will you back down from your beliefs? Will you give up hope on receiving the promise?

You do not have to live in fear if the enemy challenges your faith because your reborn spirit, created by God, is uniquely designed to overcome all challenges and obstacles. Even though Satan may try to hinder God's miracle with your name on it, you can develop the unwavering faith to face each challenge knowing without a doubt that the victory is just ahead.

Realize you find yourself in the battle, the battle is not yours, but *the battle belongs to the Lord!* If you do not have a personal relationship with Him, stop! Get that taken care of. Ask Jesus to save you. Ask Jesus to come into your heart (look in the back of this book for instructions to continue). If you truly believe, and if you ask Jesus to save you, salvation is that simple. You belong to him. He is now your spiritual Father. The victories I've been talking about will be yours at the end of the battle.

There are conduits and there are obstacles to winning the victories.

Major conduits to victories are faith in God, right thinking and right speaking. Major obstacles to victories are lack of faith, wrong thinking and wrong speaking. For instance, are you a complainer?

If we constantly complain, we will remain where we are, and the battle ends up ours instead of being in the Lord's hands. Believe right, think right and speak right!

> **Proverbs 18:21** *Death and life are in the power of the tongue; and those who love it will eat its fruit.*

Do not allow Satan to fill your mind (soul) or heart with foolish thoughts. "My husband is going to die." "No one survives cancer." "I'm going to be alone, I might as well make plans for his funeral." Put these thoughts away! Get a hold of your faith!

Jerry and I chose to speak a 'positive faith,' which is what we taught our congregation. We had preached how believers have authority over sickness and disease. Now we were living it before the people who had their eyes on us. We were now a living testimony. Do you realize without a test there is no victory? No test—no testimony!

> **Hebrews 11:6** says *But without faith it is impossible to please Him.*

God is not moved by screaming and yelling at Him. God is moved by our faith. So when Jerry sat down with me and told me what the doctor said, we agreed together at this very intense and emotional moment to trust God and lean not to our own understanding.

We certainly did not understand what was happening in our lives, but we knew from the word of God that we needed to put all of our trust in our Lord and Savior, Jesus Christ. He would be the one to help us in this time of trouble. We believed He would because He had not finished His plan for our lives. We believed God had a path for us in this situation even though we did not know where the path was leading us.

In the book of Exodus, Moses and the children of Israel fled from Egypt, and they came to the Red Sea. They became afraid and began to talk against Moses. "Why did you bring us out here to die?" **Psalms 77:19** makes it clear that God's way was in the sea, and His paths were in the mighty waters, and His footprints may not be known.

The children of Israel couldn't see it. Their faith was weak. Moses, full of faith and confidence in his God, told them to *'stand still and see the salvation of the Lord.'* We need to remember we are God's children and God is working behind the scenes on our behalf.

It may look hopeless, but trust Him. He still has a plan in place even if we don't know which way to turn, how to pray or what to believe. We must place our undivided trust in Him and His plan.

When Adam and Eve rebelled against God in the garden, sin entered into the world and disease also became part of our world, too. We also aide in our many health problems society faces today because we don't eat the right foods, we don't get enough rest for our bodies, nor do we follow proper hygiene methods like washing our hands as often as we should. Although society adds to the health conditions many of us face, there is no doubt that Satan is the root, the father of disease, the one that sends disease into the world, and wants to destroy lives with sickness in whatever manner he can use.

> *John 10:10* *The thief comes only to steal and kill and destroy; I come that they may have life, and have it more abundantly.*

If you are ever faced with a horrible sickness, do not run away from God, or think God has put this disease on you to teach you a lesson, or to humble you. Satan is the thief. He is the murderer, but God is a God of love! You wouldn't put cancer on someone you love to teach them a lesson, would you? Absolutely not! God wouldn't either. He loves us, we are His children and He wants us healthy and whole, which is His will for us. ***It is God's will to heal!***

> *3 John 1:2* *Beloved, I pray that in all respects you may prosper and be in good health, just as your soul prospers.*

Having a solid foundation in God and in His word, we read scriptures pertaining to Jerry's situation; faith based scriptures like these listed here:

> *Hebrews 13:8* *Jesus Christ is the same yesterday and today and forever.*

> *III John 1:2* *Beloved, I pray that in all respects you may prosper and be in good health, just as our soul prospers.*

> *James 1:17* *Every good thing given and every perfect gift is from above, coming down from the Father of lights, with whom there is no variation or shifting shadow.*

> *Romans 8:31* *What then shall we say to these things? If God is for us, who is against us?*

Malachi 3:6 *For I, the Lord, do not change; therefore you, O sons of Jacob, are not consumed.*

Isaiah 41:10 *Do not fear, for I am with you; Do not anxiously look about you, for I am your God. I will strengthen you, surely I will help you, surely I will uphold you with My righteous right hand.*

Numbers 23:19 *God is not a man, that He should lie, nor a son of man, that He should repent; Has He said, and will he not do it? Or has He spoken, and will he not make it good?*

Job 37:23 *The Almighty—we cannot find Him; He is exalted in power and he will not do violence to justice and abundant righteousness.*

Psalms 103:3 *Who pardons all your iniquities, Who heals all your diseases.*
There were several other Scriptures we stood in faith on.
My personal favorite Scripture I quoted constantly was:

Jeremiah 30:17 *'For I will restore you to health and I will heal you of your wounds,' declares the Lord, 'Because they have called you an outcast, saying: "It is Zion; no one cares for her."*

There were times when it looked like Jerry was dying and wouldn't make it another day, yet we were faithful to speak God's word.

We would not allow fear to rule us! Often, when people hear the diagnosis, "CANCER," fear tries to flood them. They immediately start thinking in their minds, 'I'm going to die.' 'No one survives cancer.' 'This is the end of my life.' 'This is fatal.' You see, the problem lies in the mind. That is where the battle is. Not only are you in a battle against the horrible disease in your body, you are also in a battle in your mind. You must deal with the barrage of thoughts entering at a bullet's speed at times. Fight!

When your mind is screaming pain, nausea, death, what are you saying? FIGHT! What words are coming out of your mouth?

FIGHT! Every time you vomit, you may feel one step closer to death. FIGHT against those negative thoughts running through your mind!

Those negative emotions and thoughts you're feeling exist, but you must not speak out every thought you have unless it lines up with the word of God. Your mind must be renewed to speak what the word of God says. Believe right, think right, speak right!

There were times Jerry would sit on the edge of the bed and cry, and in his mind he wanted to give up, but his heart overrode his mind because he was rooted in the word of God. Cancer can reduce the person afflicted to an insecure, dependent person. He had times of becoming so dependent on me that he wanted me near him at all times. You see, we had to fight a good fight of faith, too! Fear was trying to consume him and take control of his mind. And we knew where the fear was coming from. Satan is the author of fear!

I would be in another part of the house and Jerry would call out to me just to see where I was and if I was close by. This can be draining to the cheerleader. Sometimes you feel like you need to get away and spend some alone time because a person needs those times of refreshing and renewing. A good massage and the Word of God works wonders! However, I could feel his need and compassion would not allow me to leave him alone. Thank God for family members, as I would call them to do many errands for me When you are in the battle against cancer for several years, there are days when you fall into times of depression. We did! However, those times can be few if you stay in the word of God—with your cheerleader leading you. When Satan tries to capture you and chain you to depression, and he will, open your Bible and read it! This is where you gain control. As you read His word, your physical and mental strength will become stronger so you can continue to believe right and speak right. God's word tells us how we can build ourselves up:

> **Jude 20** *But you, beloved, building yourselves up on your most holy faith, praying in the Holy Spirit . . .*

You need a support team in place to help cheer you on. The team needs to be "on" and ready to go twenty-four seven. The team needs to be strong in the faith to be the encourager who can boldly speak the word with faith to the one who needs to hear it. I wouldn't have to encourage Jerry very long before he would snap right out of the depression. He simply needed a team member to give him hope, to give him a little nudge to get past those down times. He was my soul mate. We were joined together through our love for each other and through our love for God. It is wonderful to have a strong support system around you, cheering you on every day. Sadly, not everyone is as blessed to have people praying for them, cheering for them through all the chemo treatments, blood transfusions, platelet transfusions, bone marrow transplants, and hundreds of doctor visits. Who in their right mind wants to go through all that alone?

I tried to be there for Jerry every step of the way. Lots of nights I would stay all night in his hospital room to be company for him. I knew it made him more comfortable with me there and he would sleep better. Many times those chairs or beds were not comfortable and of course, the times of being woke up when a nurse came in to take his vital signs left us very tired. Were these times fun? Of course not. But I wouldn't have had it any other way. I loved Jerry.

Love compels one to lay down their life for one another. That time I was able to give myself completely to Jerry was such a small sacrifice on my part. If I had been in his shoes, I would want a strong cheerleader on my team to motivate me; someone strong in the faith, someone that wouldn't retreat in the heat of the battle, when the war raged during its strongest conflict. I would want someone to stand with me against Satan wearing the full armor of God, guarding me against all of his evil attacks. The enemy needs to know someone is on duty around the clock, with their guard up, and that he has no part in the picture! A good spiritual team member knows Satan is a defeated foe, that he is a loser, and will stay and fight this enemy with all that is in them.

God's word says *if you abide in me and my word abides in you, You shall ask what you will, and it shall be done for you.*

KNOWLEDGE of God's word is power, and it will set you free!

Chapter Two

If someone close to you is diagnosed with cancer, and if you truly love that person, you will be a support system to him or her. You may be the team captain, especially if you're a spouse or a parent with a child still at home. Your loved one will be counting on you to prop them up because there will be times they want to give up.

That desire doesn't usually come from their heart, but from their head. Their emotional battle could also be demonic. Pray for discernment to know how to encourage them accurately.

Cancer will definitely cause your loved one to grow weary during the battle. And they will certainly need you to be their coach, giving them the encouragement to stay in the game, and to not give in to fear or flight. They need you to encourage them to press on!

No, you don't battle cancer with literal cheers, but you will be an emotional cheerleader for them. Cheerleaders in real life practice to get their routines perfected. As a cheerleader for life and health, you will practice, practice, and practice some more. How? With the Word of God! You will read, meditate and not let it depart from your mouth.

Give them hope! Tell them the enemy (the devil) has messed with the wrong person. Cheer them on! Tell them they will make it.

The word of God is true. God is not a man that He should lie!

It is God's will for you or your loved one to be healed. Tell them they will live and not die and declare the works of the Lord. Tell them they are a fighter! Tell them they are an over comer! Tell them they can run through a troop and leap over a wall! Tell them they will win this fight and to not give up!

You can influence your loved one to change their thought pattern by your positive attitude and spirit. Take control. Be a strong force in your household. You become the lead cheerleader! Be a barrier between the enemy and your household!

From the beginning of time, Satan went to Eve to deceive her in the Garden of Eden. Why didn't he go to Adam instead? For one thing, Satan knew if he got to Eve, he would get to Adam because of the great influence she had over him. Don't underestimate your role! I kept Kenneth Hagin Sr.'s book chocked full of healing scriptures right by Jerry's bedside. I would read those scriptures over and over to him day and night. I was the head cheerleader, and I took charge! Ready to go to battle if necessary. I had strong faith, strong hope! I never ever had a strong feeling that Jerry would die.

Yes, there were times the enemy would try to put a vision in my head of Jerry in a casket at his funeral. I would quickly rebuke that and visualize Jerry behind the pulpit, strong, vibrant and preaching the word. I wouldn't give Satan an edge. That doesn't mean he won't continue to try. He will! If he can get you to continue to think, or visualize a negative thought, he will become the winner.

You cannot allow that to happen, and your loved one is counting on you to not let that happen!

> *Hebrews11:1 Faith is the assurance of things hoped for, the conviction of things not seen.*
> *Proverbs 18:21 Death and life are in the power of the tongue, and those that love it shall eat its fruit.*

Many times I would reason together with the Lord concerning the **Mark 11:24** scripture which says, *therefore I say to you, all things for which you pray and ask, believe that you have received them, and they will be granted you.* Of course, my desire was to have my husband whole. I desired one hundred percent manifestation of healing in his body. I knew he was already healed over 2000 years ago when Jesus went to the cross, now it needed to be made manifest in his body on this side of the earth!

Isaiah 53:5 *He was pierced through for our transgressions,*

He was crushed for our iniquities; The chastening for our well-being fell upon Him, and by His scourging we are healed.

Do you believe the word of God when we read it? Do I

REALLY believe the word of God when I read it? If we do, we need to follow Scripture's directions if we want to succeed on this earth. Have you or seen someone go to an owner's manual to find out how to fix something or to figure out how something is supposed to work? An owner's manual will also let you know more features that are for your ease and enjoyment if you only know it's there to use.

God's Word is our manual. It is wise for instruction!

Romans 4:17 . . . *in the presence of Him whom he believed, even God, who gives life to the dead and calls into being that which does not exist.*
I Peter 2:24 . . . *and He Himself bore our sins in His body on the cross, so that we might die to sin and live to righteousness; for by His wounds you were healed.*
John 15:7 . . . *If you abide in Me, and My words abide in you, ask whatever you wish, and it will be done for you.*
Hebrews 4:16 . . . *Therefore let us draw near with confidence to the throne of grace, so that we may receive mercy and find grace to help in time of need.*

Jerry spent two years in remission, then the cancer returned more aggressive than the first time. He made an appointment with his doctor and was told he needed a bone marrow transplant.

Because of his age, they would use his own bone marrow and not need a donor. We decided to get a second opinion. The second doctor concurred and set up an appointment with another doctor in Kansas City. My husband had to go through a series of tests to see if he would be eligible to be a candidate for a transplant.

Uprooting was not easy, but thank the Lord, all of our children lived in the Kansas City area so we would have a place to stay.

We would also have the support of all ten of our children, twenty- five grandchildren, and thirteen great grandchildren.

We packed for several months, made arrangements for someone to take care of our church congregation in Beardstown, Illinois, and off to Kansas City we went. Jerry was admitted directly into the Kansas University Medical Center Hospital. He went through a series of tests for fourteen days. Dr. Deauna said, "Mr. Houchins, you have Lymphoma Cancer, but it is doable. If you are going to get cancer, this is the one to get. We can cure this!"

CHAPTER THREE

The Treatment Begins

Our previous battle was hard enough, but we were really in it now.

Jerry went through several months of the strongest chemotherapy called R.I.C.E. In January, 2008, he was ready for the Bone Marrow Transplant.

They harvested his own stem cells from his marrow and froze it, then they gave him a week of very strong chemo. After this, they thawed his stem cells and injected them back into his body.

During this time, all cancer cells and his own immune system were destroyed.

We were able to come home from the hospital, and two days later, around two a.m., I tried to wake him to take some medicine, and he did not respond. We had to call the ambulance, and they took him back to the hospital. He had gone into septic shock.

They did not expect him to live to morning. He was closer to death than life.

At first, the medics were barely able to find his blood pressure.

Later, he became stable enough to go to the intensive care unit.

He was put on oxygen. They doctors found that he had an infection, but they did not know the cause of it, so they were giving him up to fifteen bags of medicine at one time.

A heart doctor was called in because they were positive the infection was causing his heart to beat 170 BPM (beats per minute). The physician indicated we needed to induce him into a coma, put him on a ventilator, and shock his heart to get it to come back into rhythm. We both agreed to the procedure.

Our children were there, and we all gathered around his bed to pray. He wanted us to read one of his favorite scriptures out of Psalm 23. Some of his children did not understand our strong faith, and began to get nervous, obviously thinking he was preparing to die. NO! He was preparing to live!

The medical staff did the procedure and his heart responded, coming down to 99 to 110 BPM, which made the doctor happy.

There were two doctors coming and going. I called them Dr.

Negative and Dr. Positive. Dr. Negative came into the room and said, "I am so sorry we can't do more for your husband."

I said, "Excuse me, what do you mean?"

"What does your husband do for a living?"

"He's a minister."

"Oh, he won't be able to do that any longer, he has congestive heart failure. He will need a defibrillator, a wheelchair and oxygen with him at all times. He will not be able to climb stairs, or ever return to work."

He turned to walk out of the room and this cheerleader sprang into action! How dare he be so presumptuous to speak those negative things, leaving little hope? He didn't know how Jerry would respond to medical treatment. I began to quote the word of God!

The word of God says to *pull down every evil imagination that exalts itself above the knowledge of God.* I began to pull down every negative word and evil imagination Dr. Negative spoke that landed on me, and on Jerry!

"Satan, you are liar, and I do not receive this negative report.

I do not believe any diagnosis of congestive heart failure, I pull down every one of those negative words that were just planted in this room," I responded. Whose report was I going to believe?

There was no question about it I was going to believe God's report, and so was Jerry!

Am I going to believe Dr. Negative or am I going to believe

I Peter 2:24 which says, *"by the stripes of Jesus I am healed"*?

I truly believed by the stripes of Jesus my husband is healed and was healed! I truly believed Jesus nailed *all* our diseases to the Cross thousands of years ago. And I truly believed Jerry was redeemed from all disease, and that it had no legal right to be in his body!

I went from the encouraging cheerleader to being a warrior. He could not fight for himself, he was in a coma. I had to fight! I had to counter attack the words Dr. Negative had spoken! I did not want those negative words to affect my husband's path in any way.

We had a Jewish Prayer Shawl (Tallit) spread out over his bed.

Sometimes the nurses would put it in his drawer, and I would get it back out and put it back on his bed. Do you know when Jairus's daughter was sick unto death, it was the Jewish custom to wrap the ill in the Tallit? Jairus wrapped his daughter in the Tallit, having no doubt she would be healed. When Jesus arrived on the scene, He said, "Tabitha, wrapped in the Tallit, come forth," and she was raised from the dead! Is God a respecter of persons? No!

The Bible says He isn't, and I had no doubt my husband was going to rise up off his bed totally healed before my eyes.

As I was speaking the scriptures over Jerry, our Pastor, Pastor Gary Kruzan, and Reverend Billy Miller, both from Illinois, walked into the room. They had driven three hundred miles just to visit and pray for Jerry. That's what the body of Christ looks like! That's what love looks like!

Pastor Gary said, "What are you doing?" I said "Come into the hall."

"Pastor, I am drawing a blood line around Jerry."

Then I proceeded to tell him what Dr. Negative had spoke over Jerry. Jerry had a good relationship with Pastor Gary, and had shared with him the scriptures we were standing on. He had one of his prayer captains type them up, then they were distributed to the congregation so we would all be united in our prayers. Pastor Gary had those typed out scriptures with him and read them over Jerry.

Then we prayed over him while he was still in the coma.

The next day, Dr. Positive came in to see Jerry. He was so excited to see the progress Jerry had made. I asked him if there was going to be any damage to Jerry's heart after what he had experienced, and he said, "I believe he's going to be fine. He has a very strong heart and should live a normal life. It's a good report Ms. Houchins"

WHAT! Do we believe Dr. Negative? Or do we believe the good report of God's Word, and Dr. Positive's words? That was a no-brainer for us! What if I had simply believed Dr. Negative?

Would things have turned out different? I have no doubt because death and life are in the power of the tongue! Yes, we may slip and say something negative from time—to-time, but realize when we do, we have planted a seed and will reap a harvest if we let it go. It's never to late to repent. Be quick to reverse those doubt filled words by replacing them with positive **faith words.**

Words spoken, either positive or negative will produce a harvest.

That's why it's so important to watch what we believe, what we think, and what we speak!

Where Dr. Negative tried to dash my hope, Dr. Postive rebuilt it.

After an Electro-cardiogram and Echo-cardiogram was ran, they showed Jerry's heart 100% strong. The technician even commented how strong the walls of Jerry's heart were after all the chemo he had taken.

After hearing a good report, I'm feeling victorious. Satan has been defeated another round, and when that happens, it makes you feel you could burst out in praise, and I did!

We were basking in the glorious victory of winning another round for the glory of God, full of hope, knowing all is going to be fine!

Then a whole team of doctors come into the room only to knock the wind right out of my sails.

One of the surgeons said, "Mrs. Houchins do you have a power of attorney?"

"Yes, I do, why?"

"Your husband's scan showed a cloudiness over his bowels, and we think his small bowel is dead. I need to do exploratory surgery to make sure, and need to do that right now. I will open him up to check him, and if necessary, I may come out to talk to you to see how aggressive you want me to be. It may be that we only need to remove his small bowel. If all his bowels are dead, we will close him up and just make him comfortable. We will need you to sign these permission papers for the surgery on his behalf."

If you are not full of the word of God, and on that emotional roller coaster many people are on, **you will fall apart!** Without the word of God there is no foundation to hold you up. You emotions will take control of you, and you will feel like collapsing to the floor.

After hearing this news, let's be honest. This cheerleader now needed encouraged! Thankfully, my daughter was there to put her arms around me and hug me while many emotions were flooding my mind.

I felt like everyone else was in control of this crises for a moment.

I realized this was a test on my part, and I would quickly find out if my faith in God was really in my heart or just in my head. Were my words of faith I'd been speaking simply to impress my peers?

We quickly find out what we're made of in the heat of the battle!

The children left the room and shut the door so I could have a few moments alone with Jerry. Still in the coma, unaware of what was about to happen to him, he could offer no advice, guidance, comfort or assurance.

I pulled myself together and began to talk to him as if he were awake.

All of a sudden I felt a whoosh of air brush my back side. I thought it was a nurse coming into the room to prepare Jerry for surgery. I moved away from the bed, looked around and the room was empty.

I sensed by the Holy Spirit I had just been brushed by an angel.

Angels minister to the heirs of salvation, and I had no doubt they were in the room attending to God's business. A peace came over me, and I felt in control again. I knew in my heart he would survive and it would not be as the surgeon had said. I signed the papers.

Even though I sensed a calmness inside, sometimes the heart and the head doesn't connect at the same time. Another doctor came in and I asked, "He seems so weak, am I making the right decision? Is he able to survive this surgery?"

The doctor replied, "When he came to the emergency room, he was very fragile, and he would not have survived. If we wait, he will not live. You have a small window of opportunity right now, and he has the best chance of surviving. You have definitely made the right decision." Our family gathered in the surgery waiting room as he was taken into surgery. Four hours later, the doctor came out with a big smile on his face. He told us his bowels were fine but his gall bladder looked bad and he removed it. Jerry started making progress immediately. His breathing and vital signs returned to normal. Or normal for him . . . he always had very low blood pressure.

The next step the doctors took was to bring Jerry out of the coma.

They quit giving him the meds that had kept him asleep. Three days later, there was concern because he was not responding. The devil was still trying to interfere. That's what he does . . . steal, kill and destroy. The enemy knew I was emotionally and physically worn down from being at Jerry's bedside for five days straight, and probably figured he had the upper hand, but he did not! Of course, he continued trying to work on my emotions, continued to try and put fear on me with thoughts like, "Your husband is not coming out of the coma." "He may be in that coma for years, you've heard of that haven't you?" "He is going to die!"

"SHUT UP DEVIL!" I said.

"He shall live and not die and will decree and declare the works of the Lord!"

Satan never gives up *until* you tell him to shut up. No matter how exhausted you may become, the word of God is still alive in you, sharper than any two-edged sword, fully able to defeat the enemy of God. Yes, it is true . . . you can become spiritually weak in this type of situation, but all you have to do is open your Bible, read several powerful passages of scripture to come out of whatever it is you are feeling. Spiritual strength is re-newed!

> *Romans 8:31.* . . *If God be for us, who can be against us.*
> *Malachi 3:6.* . . *For I, the Lord, do not change.*

I read this scripture to Jerry and said, "Jerry, your health is going to spring forth speedily!"

He squeezed my hand!

> *Isaiah 58:8.* . . *Then your light will break out like the dawn, and your recovery will speedily spring forth; and your righteousness will go before you; the glory of the Lord will be your rear guard.*

I read another one of his favorite scriptures and afterwards, **he slightly nodded his head!**

Isaiah 41:10. . . do not fear, for I am with you; do not anxiously look about you for I am your God. I will strengthen you, surely I will help you, surely I will uphold you with My righteous right hand.

I was getting pretty excited at this point. Tears began to form in the corner of my eyes I said, "Jerry, the scripture says you will not die, but you shall live and declare and decree the works of the Lord!

Many people need to hear your story. People living without hope- need to hear your testimony!"

He opened his eyes.

What a welcome sight to look into those big, hazel/green eyes! He was a mess physically. No hair anywhere on his body, one hundred forty-six pounds of nothing but skin and bones, so weak he couldn't hold a cup. I didn't care—I loved him!

CHAPTER 4

Faith Tested

There was nothing masculine about him, but I didn't care. I was so excited to see him with his eyes open! He was my hero, my husband, my friend, my pastor. I only seen him as the man I deeply loved.

The first night Jerry was conscious, his daughter, Angela, sat all night with him to allow me some rest. He had been closer to death than anyone I had ever known and made it back, and beginning his journey back to health, ready to experience wellness, living life abundantly like the scripture promises.

The ventilator and heart monitor were removed. After forty days (of being in the wilderness), he was released from the hospital, and we were on our way back home to Illinois! Jerry had lost over sixty pounds, lost all of his hair, and lost most of his strength, but he never once lost the victory!

On the less than positive side, he became very dependent on me.

Cancer is a definite thief, just like our spiritual enemy! It robs the person of life as they knew it before. He had to continue to receive blood and platelet transfusions. Overcoming the dreaded disease consumes both lives of the team captain and the cheerleader.

Your lives revolve around going to the Cancer Treatment Center, and fighting a war against an unseen enemy. Just like the devil, you can't see him, but you know he's there.

Ten hour days were spent at the medical center day after day.

You have no time for yourself. It robs you of finances. Every penny you may have in your savings goes for medical expenses.

Even after dealing with all these negative things, Jerry never retreated. Yes, he had some down moments, but I never heard him say, "I'm done. I can't go another day. It's not worth it." He was the strongest man of faith I have ever known.

Certainly there were times when he looked like he would not make it, but we did not base our faith on our feelings or what things looked like. Circumstances change; however, prayer changes circumstances. Our faith and confidence were in God and in His word.

While we were in Kansas, our church went on just as if we were there. Our Pastor friend became an overseer on our behalf. The church body went to his services on Sunday, and we ordained a lady in the church to the helps ministry to hold the Wednesday night Bible Study. The church continued to support us with finances (which we were blessed to be able to give back), cards, and prayers.

Jerry had always handled the finances in our personal lives, and worked with the church secretary with the finances in the church.

I would now have to accept that responsibility. I stayed in contact with the church secretary, telling her which bills to pay each week, and sometimes I would make several trips to Illinois to handle problems that would arise. Overall, we were very thankful and blessed to have such a great congregation. They stood together, worked together, and prayed through the adverse situation of not having their Pastor there to help them with their own personal problems. We knew it wasn't easy for some of them, and fully understood why they felt the need to go to other churches. This battle touched many people.

Pastor Kruzan supported us in many ways, too. Besides coming to Kansas to be with Jerry to pray for him, he became overseer of our church, and each month his own church sent money to help with expenses. What a blessing this was to us, as it removed a heavy burden of having to be concerned about how bills were going to get paid.

No matter what we had been through, we still believed it is God's will for Jerry to be healed, and continued to stand on the scripture *3 John 2 Beloved, I wish above all things that you may prosper and be in health, even as your soul prospers.*

When you are Pastors of a church and someone comes up for prayer, it is easy to lay hands on them and pray the prayer of faith.

However, the pressure is on when the sickness is in your own body.

If you did not know what the Bible says about healing, and understand the fact that it belongs to you, you may never enter into that complete manifestation of healing.

This may sound somewhat confusing when I say you are healed, and then you need to receive your healing. Receiving your healing through the prayer of faith is asking God for something in the name of Jesus.

When you ask for healing in prayer, you *must believe* you have received it by faith, even if you're still sick! We cannot be controlled by our five senses. The Bible instructs us in **II Corinthians 5:7** to *"walk by faith and not by sight."* This is not easy to do at times.

When Jerry was vomiting and having to go to the bathroom, it's hard to believe you're healed! When the doctor gives you that bad report as we had been given many times, it's hard to continue to believe. I said earlier, this battle is in the mind, and must be controlled and subjected to the Word of God.

There is a scripture Joyce Meyer uses quite often that really fits here:

> *II Corinthians 10: 4-5* . . . *for the weapons of our warfare are not flesh, but divinely powerful for the destruction of fortresses. We are destroying speculations and every lofty things raised up against the knowledge of God, and we are taking every thought captive to the obedience of Christ.*

The word says to cast down all thoughts and imaginations that are contrary to the promises in God's Word.

Faith comes from God's Word. Faith comes from hearing God's word. Faith is a gift of God so no one can boast about anything but Him! When you read God's word aloud, your ears are hearing Who do you believe the most—yourself! Therefore, when you hear yourself say, "By His stripes I am healed," you begin to believe in your heart and your body responds to what you're saying. When you are praying the prayer of faith, and hearing what your mouth is saying, it will come to pass. An IMPORTANT note: Our prayer must be the "prayer of faith," and not the "prayer from the head." When you're praying the right prayer, you're standing on the word of God, and healing will come.

When Christians begin to stand in faith, the temptation is there to try and work up things. For example, even as an adult Christian, Jerry would try to "work up his healing." He would say things like, "Maybe there is something I am not doing." "Maybe there is something else I need to do." You cannot work for your healing . . . you can believe right, think right, speak right.

Forgiveness is also CRUCIAL to getting our prayers answered.

In *Mark 11:25-26*, we are commanded to forgive if we have aught against anybody. No hate, resentment, animosity, or dislike against anyone is permissible where God is concerned! If we want forgiven we must forgive. Don't put it off for another second! The devil will use these things to hinder your prayers.

Through self-examination, and asking God to forgive us, our hearts will be cleansed from anything that may stop our healing.

Forgiveness is a powerful tool given to us from God. Use it!

We believe we had done everything we knew to do. We were in relationship with our Father, we believed in Him, we were committed to His word. We were determined to walk in forgiveness. We were determined to believe right, to think right, and speak right to the best of our ability. Sure, we had our share of crying, feeling discouraged, but we were determined to not allow our emotions to rule us. No matter what Jerry's body was screaming against him, or no matter what Dr. Negative was speaking against Him, we were determined to believe and confess God's report, which is a good one!

I will say it again because we believe this with every fiber of our being: when it comes to the body being healed from cancer or any other disease, the word of God must be on our tongue!

Proverbs 18:21 *Death and life are in the power of the tongue, and they that love it shall eat its fruit.*

From the beginning of time the devil has messed with our language.

He has helped us speak sentences about death. How many times do we say these phrases such as 'That scared me to death!' 'I was frightened to death!' 'I thought I was going to die!' 'I could have died!' 'I love them to death!' 'That was to die for!' My feet (or) head is killing me!

We use the word *death* or *die* so casually, without realizing our ears are hearing that word and planting seeds of death in our spirit! It is a clever device of Satan to slip destructive words into our vocabulary.

Interesting why we don't we use the word *life* instead of *death?*

It is definitely not easy to change after a lifetime of saying those phrases. It takes concentration. Jerry and I had a little game we played. When he would make a negative statement, I would say, "Well, if that's what you want to come to pass, then just keep confessing that." We would laugh and call ourselves the "Word Gestapo!"

Heading back home to Illinois in April, 2007, we knew we had to continually be on guard to what we spoke out of our mouths. When we arrive home, we resumed as pastors of our church. Jerry was not yet strong enough to preach so I would preach in his place. Of course, he wanted to do something, so he would open the service and do some of the preliminaries. On Father's Day, he was able to resume the duties of Pastor and I returned to teaching the toddler class.

My husband was still getting approximately four units of blood and two units of platelets twice a week because of the trauma he had suffered going through gall bladder surgery. That was hardly anything compared to what we'd been through, and we were so thankful it seemed things were getting back to normal.

One night he suddenly took ill running a high temperature. Back to the emergency room we went. He had double pneumonia, and they did not think he would make it through the day. They began to pump him full of antibiotics, put a chest tube in to drain his lungs and gave him oxygen to help him breathe. He contacted MRSA, a bacterial infection that is highly resistant to some antibiotics, and had to be put in isolation. I had to wear a gown, gloves, and mask, as well as anyone else who entered the room.

They decided to do an endoscope and found pea size nodules in his small intestine that were oozing blood. They decided not to correct it at this time. Jerry left the hospital twenty-one days later, and was back preaching in the pulpit once again.

One Sunday morning I was in my classroom and one of the ladies in the church came in and said, "Pastor Marge come quick, Pastor Jerry passed out and is very ill." I got to the sanctuary as fast as I could. He had been sitting on a tall stool preaching when he suddenly got quite ill and vomited all over the pulpit and became extremely weak.

Three of the men took him home, and stayed with him while I took over the pulpit to preach a message in Jerry's place. I was thankful the Holy Spirit gave me the strength needed to control my emotions, and yet, that morning was the catalyst that made us realize we were not going to be able to continue in the ministry.

Jerry needed to return to Kansas City for further treatment. We made plans to make the move there for good. Our children came to Illinois and helped us prepare for a huge auction. This was one of the hardest things we had encountered in our marriage life together. We had a lot of ties to the Beardstown community.

We were living our dream, ministering in this church for the past eight years, we were attached to the people there.

They were not happy about us leaving either, but wanted the best for their Pastors. We had to sell almost everything we owned, including our home. The good thing in all this was the fact we were going to be with our nine children, twenty—five grand children and thirteen great grand-children.

Thinking about moving near our family caused us to reflect on November, 2006, when our thirty-three year old daughter, Melinda, was killed in a car accident. She wouldn't be with us in Kansas, but we tried to think on the positive end of things . . . she was an organ donor and helped over seventy-five people with her organs and tissue. She also left behind four children. The urgency increased to be with our family after her death, and now it was coming to fruition.

Our former Pastor agreed to take over our ministry we were leaving behind, and since his church was only sixteen miles away, it worked out well for everyone. The transfer took only several months to complete. The people had been going to his church for eight months when we gone before, so they were already making adjustments. Some would not agree to make Rushville the location for their new church home and would find new places of worship.

The ones that decided to make the congregation in Rushville their church home have fit in wonderfully, and are continuing in their ministries to be a blessing in that assembly.

Pastor Kruzan, in the beginning stages, turned our facility into a children's ministry. There were anywhere between fifty and seventy-five children ministered to every Thursday night, and many have been saved, and more people have been added to his church because of the transition that took place. We are so thankful how God worked it all out.

We sold our home in one week. That was a God thing with the economy so slow, the market not moving, and so many foreclosures.

We were blessed to get top price for our house! God worked miracles! Our children came and moved us to Kansas. We put our things in storage and lived with our oldest daughter and son-in- law for eight months before finding a home.

During this time, Jerry was feeling worse, and needed to return to his original doctor. She could not believe how sickly he was. He was white as a sheet, weighing only 147 pounds. He was weak from the loss of blood. She admitted him into the hospital after checking him over. His blood pressure was 70/40. His hemoglobin count was five (normal range is 13.5 to 16.50). His platelet count was 16,000 (normal range is 150,000 to 400,000).

They gave him eight units of blood over the next few days and six units of platelets. They ran five endoscopes trying to find the cause of the bleed problem.

Her first words were, "It is my gut feeling the Lymphoma is back."

We could not believe she would make a statement like this without getting the results from the tests she had ordered. We had to go to battle again, confessing the Word, rebuking the negative words! After more tests, she came back to Jerry's room and said, "Mr. Houchins, I don't think I will be able to fix you this time.

Where would you like to die? You can die in the hospital, in a hospice facility or at home. You can give this some thought, talk to your wife and let me know."

The next day her assistant came in to talk to me. We had come here for healing and they were telling us he is going to die! Later in the morning, a social worker came in to discuss the arrangements.

We listened to what he had to say, then Jerry spoke up. "Sir, I have patiently listened to you and now you listen to me. I did not come here to die. I have been at death's door twice and I am not ready to die." He continued, "**Psalm 91:1** says *He that dwells in the secret place of the most High shall abide under the shadow of the Almighty.* The word Almighty throughout the Old Testament means El Shaddai. This means God is more than enough, the God of impossibilities."

He wasn't done speaking. "Right here in this hospital in January, 2006, I received a bone marrow transplant. After that, I went into septic shock and they thought I was dying. They did exploratory surgery and found an infected gall bladder. They didn't think I would live through the night. I was here in this hospital for forty days. El Shaddai, the God of impossibilities brought me through that. Then in September, 2007, at Springfield Memorial Hospital, I was admitted with double pneumonia. I was there for twenty-one days. Once again they didn't think I would live through the day.

El Shaddai brought me through that. He's the God of impossibilities! Jesus said in the New Testament that what is impossible with man is possible with God. So I am going to live. I didn't come here to die, but to live and declare the works of the Lord. I have confidence that El Shaddai will bring me through this!"

The social worker choked up a bit and said, "Mr. Houchins, maybe we are having this conversation prematurely. I can see you are a man of great faith."

Then he excused himself and left the room. I said, "WOW, Jerry, that was quite a sermon you preached to that man." We both felt peace. And even though there was a mutual respect, the medical professionals still felt they had done all they could do.

Maybe they had, but we weren't finished. We were still holding on!

We went to see Dr. Mark Wallace, Jerry's chiropractor, and we told him our ongoing situation. He consulted with other colleagues about Jerry's case, and they came up with an herb mixture they wanted Jerry to try.

He said, "Jerry I would like for you to take this herb mixture. It is guaranteed to stop the bleeding."

We remembered a prophetic word Dr. Ron Smith had given us from the Lord. "The right person needs to get their hands on you."

Two weeks after he started taking the herb mixture (which he said tasted awful), we began to notice a difference. His stools had improved noticeably. We went for his transfusion and they said "Mr. Houchins, you don't need anything today." This was a history making day! A day we had believed for seventeen months! The bleeding had completely stopped. The number seventeen in Bible Numerology means, 'complete victory.' He never had to have another transfusion. El Shaddai, the God of impossibilities, had given Jerry his miracle. He was cancer free, and the bleeding had stopped. My cheerleading career had ended.

There was no need for any more cheers, as we had won the game!

If you're facing an impossible situation, and you can not see your way out, or you're so discouraged to the point you feel you are ready to quit, I have seven words that can change everything.

Seven words, if you will believe them, will turn defeat into the most glorious opportunity for victory you have ever known.

'YOU ARE A CANDIDATE FOR A MIRACLE!'

If you are in Christ, you can expect God to do the impossible for you. Every challenge you face today was already overcome by Jesus over two-thousand years ago. By those stripes Jesus took, we are healed. He *paid the price to heal every sickness and disease*. Because of Him there's an answer that is older than any problem you might face. If you have cancer, diabetes, high blood pressure, heart trouble, whatever it may be, *'you are a candidate for a miracle.'*

Chapter Five

Marge's Journal

Jerry had been in the fight of his life. As Christians, we are to fight the good fight of faith! And fights are not always easy, but in God, we know they're good ones because His word says so.

When we become a Christian, we enter into a relationship with God by believing in Jesus Christ. We don't "stop" the minute we ask Jesus to save us, we keep growing, we begin reading the word of God, and continue to do so until we die. We learn to pray, and continue to pray until we die. Faith is definitely a gift of God, lest any one should boast, but our faith is to grow, and that's a decision each person has to make.

Each time we see a Scripture we've read work, that builds our faith, too! The word of God is full of wonderful promises. We have to find out what they are. If we continue to pray, we will see God move on our behalf and answer our prayers. Each answer to prayer encourages us to keep praying! It also teaches us God loves us, and we learn to trust God more and more.

Experiences in life are the best teachers. Before we became pastors we owned a Heating, Cooling and Electrical company. I remember a time when we had a Loan on Equipment coming due. We had already extended it once and the company was in some financial distress and did not want to give us another extension. We held hands and prayed for direction and agreed together that God would help us out.

We had a beautiful black stallion horse "Pearls Black George" that had won the 1999 "World Grand Championship" in Ava, Mo.

Jerry decided to try to sell him to pay the note. He called a man that had bought several horses from us and offered George to him.

He said he would love to buy him but Jerry needed to convince his wife. Upon approaching her she would not even hear of it-she left the room totally against the sale. So should we give up on that idea?

We prayed again-and then waited a few days. Jerry called them again and set up a meeting to talk to him and his wife together. After Jerry talked to them about the gentleness of the stallion, the wife said they would talk it over and he should call at nine o'clock that night for their answer. The rest is history, they bought the horse, we paid the note. Everyone was happy and we had an experience we would always remember how good and faithful our God is!

When we first come to Christ, we have no idea of all the things He will do for us because we don't really have any idea of who we are in Christ. The Holy Spirit has produced sons and daughters, you and me! The Bible says sons and daughters (the believers) are adopted into the family of God, with God being our spiritual heavenly Father. The word Abba is heard in certain Christian churches, and "Abba" actually means daddy, father.

> **Romans 8:15** *For you have not received a spirit of slavery leading to fear again, but you have received a spirit of adoption as sons by which we cry out, "Abba! Father!"*

There's so much to experience for the believer if you don't refuse to grow. You do not know what your future holds. You do not know when you may need the wisdom that comes from growing in Christ.

You may find yourself in the battle for the life of a loved one, or even for your very own life. That is not the time to decide to grow up in Christ. There may be times that you will need fortitude and great spiritual strength to make it through the trial! If you're new in the Lord, I hope you won't resist as the Holy Spirit begins to draw you into a deeper relationship with the Father. The trials in life are hard enough for someone strong in faith, but a young believer or one who has not allowed themselves to grow would possibly struggle much more because they haven't learned to exercise their faith, and they wouldn't truly know the power of their God, and possibly not realize the will of God, which is crucial to fighting any battle.

> **Joshua 1:8** *This book of the law shall not depart from your mouth, but you shall meditate on it day and night, so that you may be careful to do according to all that is written in it; for then you will make your way prosperous, and then you will have success.*

To be successful, the word of God must become a truth in your spirit man, and sometimes it takes reading it over and over, meditating on it day and night, speaking it out loud. Not all truth come easily. Maybe to the head, but not to the spirit. Don't let the book of the law depart from your mouth the word of God says. In other words, keep saying it and saying it.

When you are disciplined about learning God's word, THEN the words that come out of your heart will be positive words mixed with faith. You'll quit complaining about your sickness, or the doctor's care of you, or the hospital's lack of care. As you learn the truths of God's word, you will only say what His word tells you to say. The word teaches you how to speak.

I was reading through my journal and I found the following notes:

- 1-16-06 Much has happened since my last entry. Our daughter
- Melinda was in a car accident and we had to make the decision to take her off of life support. She went home to be with the
- Lord in November 2005.
- I rolled my car on slick ice in which I did not even get a scratch.
- I was protected by the hand of the Lord.
- Ten members (one family) have moved away to another town and have left our church.
- It has been confirmed, Jerry has Lymphoma, Cancer and needs a
- Bone Marrow Transplant.
- Our daughter Gale had to have surgery.
- Friday . . . woke up in the night with a scratchy throat and a rash all over my body. Nerves are trying to take control of my body.
- I need to get into that secret place with God. I have gotten my
- Bible and have turned to Psalm 91. I need rest in the Almighty.
- All my attention has been focused on Jerry. I need a lift.

End of Entry

I know there were many days Jerry did not feel like getting out of bed, but he always made an effort to get up, get dressed and sit in his chair in the living area. The man or woman of faith realizes God is good, and that any symptoms will not prevail in their body. They will continue speaking the word. "I am victorious! I will win! Satan is a loser once again!" Even on the days he was at his worst, you could hear him saying, "Father, I thank you that my strength is being renewed as an eagle."

There were times when the devil would bring on one of his attacks, and we would burst out in laughter. Not because it was funny, but to let the enemy know he was not going to get the upper hand.

We'd remind him, "Devil, you don't have a legal right to put sick- ness on him. Sickness came because of the curse and we're not under the curse. We are redeemed! Now get out of here with your sickness, we reject you in Jesus name!"

Each time he was under attack, we would plead the blood of Jesus, quick to take authority over all sickness trying to ravage his body, and he would begin to feel better. If you don't have a support team in place, find a good faith based church, one that speaks the word and connect with them. Your church family will be on your side, cheering you on to victory!

The battle against cancer has an affect on the whole family. There are many changes that happen when living with a serious illness in the home. Lifestyle changes have to be made which can be very distressing. Daily routines may have to be adjusted to accommodate treatment schedules. The spouse tends to neglect themselves, some- times getting rattled. Many times, the one with cancer questions their identity and self worth. Sensitivity about appearance arises.

These feelings are common and may affect one's relationship with others, including sexual intimacy with their spouse. Open, honest communication regarding fears and concerns is important.

Entry in Journal:

It seems we are going through a personal struggle with each other.

I genuinely realize it is because we are under a tremendous amount of stress which has caused me to have a lot of anger, resentment, disappointment and even hardness of heart towards Jerry. We cannot allow Satan to attack us this way. He would like to divide so he can conquer. We cannot have an attitude of individualistic thoughts of 'He can live his life and I can live mine.' There's a price to pay when we have that independent spirit. There has to be more open communication, more oneness. I need more compassion.

> *I Corinthians 11:11-12 However, in the Lord, neither is woman independent of man, nor is the man independent of woman. 12 For as the woman originates from the man, so also the man has his birth through the woman; and all things originate from God.*

I must pray: Lord, nothing in me wants to pray for my husband. I am angry with him. He hurts my feelings at times and I have become a hateful, resentful, unforgiving woman. Now I surrender this all to you, Jesus. I need Your help to release these things. I need a clean heart and a right spirit before You and towards my husband. Give me a new, positive, joyful, loving, forgiving attitude toward him.

Where he has made mistakes reveal them to him and convict his heart about those things. Lead him through the path of repentance and deliverance.

Help me not to hold myself apart from him emotionally, mentally or physically because of unforgiveness. Where either of us needs to ask forgiveness of the other, help us to do so. If there is something I'm not seeing that is adding to this problem, reveal it to me and help me to understand it and make it right. Remove any wedge of confusion that has created misunderstanding or miscommunication.

Where there is behavior that needs to change in either of us, I pray you will enable that change to happen. As much as I want to hang on to my anger toward him because I feel it is justified, I want to do what is right. I release all those feelings to you. Give me a renewed love and compassion toward him and words to heal this situation."

After this prayer, I started reading Stormie O'Martian's* book, *The Power of a Praying Wife *.'* This was just what I needed, as it opened my eyes about 'me.' I had become weary because I was feeling so much stress. With the help of the book, appropriate changes began taking place in my life, and I knew how to begin praying for my husband God's way, not my way.

I respected the ministry of Pastor Joel Osteen, so I also decided to send an email and asked him how he coped with his mother's cancer.

He wrote me back and said, "Don't try to carry it alone. Turn it all over to Jesus and let Him bear the load." How simple! I was trying to bear this burden all alone.

I had Jesus in my life, but I 'needed' Jesus. Once I released it all to Jesus, I felt inner peace come into my heart and mind. Jerry and I began to have a closer relationship than we ever had. We learned we were in this 'together,' though he was the one with the cancer.

We learned to have more compassion for each other—we were both going through this experience.

If you are facing a similar situation as we did, and you don't know what to do, I would encourage you to look at **Psalm 77:14-19**. This passage talks about Moses and the children of Israel when they were fleeing from the Egyptians, and came up to the Red Sea. It says in verse 19 . . . *Your way was in the sea and Your paths in the mighty waters, and Your footprints may not be known.*

The path didn't appear all of a sudden, it was there all the time.

God was working behind the scenes on their behalf. He had prepared this path from the beginning of time for this very time of need. Although the children of Israel couldn't see it, the path was there. God has a path for every one of us. You can be assured, He has a way out of every problem you face today.

He was not going to let the people perish after delivering them from bondage. Now what this says to me is this—God is always working behind the scenes. Even when we can't see anything happening.

Even when we can't feel anything. Even when it looks the darkest, God is working on our behalf.

For the past several years, there were times when I felt I couldn't go any further, and I would remind myself God is working behind the scenes, and this situation I was in would change. If I did not truly believe that, I would not have been able to endure the trial.

If you will be sensitive to the Holy Spirit, you will discover that path.

When Israel got to the Red Sea, it looked as though it was all over.

How many times in our lives have we reached a place where we thought it is all over? The doctor has told you, "It's an impossible situation. There is no hope. Where do you want to die?"

The devil says, "This is as far as you are going." If you listen to that and dwell on the lies, they will build a *stronghold* in your mind, and you will begin to believe it.

Each one of us have negative thoughts, but the child of God walking by faith won't dwell on them to prevent strongholds from settling in their mind. The believer learns to cast down the negative thoughts even though they are facing a mountain of problems. The path of God might not be clear at certain times. The temptation is there to get so caught up in the problem that sometimes we cannot hear the Holy Spirit's direction, desiring to lead us to the path God has for us.

Yes, the battle is vicious at times, but great victories come out of great battles, and Jerry and I experienced them! Yes, we could have listened to Satan many times. I could have accepted the doctor's reports and simply said, "I just can't see any way out of this." I truly believe that statement is inspired by the devil! When God says *there's a path that runs through it*, who are we going to believe? The negative report or the positive report? There is a way even when it does not look like there is any way.

God is gracious and gives us hope, telling us just because we do not see a path doesn't mean it's not there. You may say, "I just cannot see it." Since when did you gain the ability to govern your life by what you see? God's word says *we walk by faith and not by sight!*

Obtaining victories is why the knowledge of the word is so important. You have to have the word in your heart. He has give you authority to take control over everything Satan throws your way. Choose to speak the positive **faith** God has given you, and let nothing else come out of your mouth, remembering that *death and life are in the power of the tongue.*

You will know what is in you or is not in you when you're in the heat of the battle by what words are coming out of your mouth.

The word of God is clear when it says *out of the abundance of the heart the mouth speaks.* Listen to yourself. Everyone else is listening, too, including the enemy. Keep your heart pure by filling it with the word of God. Spend enormous time with the Heavenly Father in prayer.

Matthew 12:34 *. . . out of the abundance of the heart the mouth speaks.*

Things would be much different today had we listened to Satan.

But we chose to find the path God had prepared for us. It is God's will for all to be healed. We can walk in it, believe it and receive it.

The key:

Walk in faith, walk in relationship with your heavenly Father, believe when you pray you receive, and it will come to pass!

CHAPTER SIX

Captain of the Team Departs

On February 3, 2009, Reverend Jerry Houchins, Captain of the Houchins team departed earth on his journey to "A Place Called Heaven."* He fought a good fight of faith; therefore, he had waiting for him a crown of new life once he arrived in heaven.

The last months of his life was a beautiful period of time compared to the last six year's battle he bravely faced head on. He was getting stronger. He was helping to remodel the new home we had purchased. We were experiencing such a miraculous change. It was as if he'd never had cancer.

He was in remission and had began to travel and preach once again.

That was his passion. The very last church he ministered in, he asked at the end of the service if there was anyone that needed healing. A young couple came forward and said they had been to three doctors, and was told that the wife could never conceive or deliver a baby. Rev. Jerry spoke faith into the couple and then asked them if they could put their faith out there and believe for her to be healed. Their answer was a firm yes. He laid hands on them and prayed the prayer of faith.

It wasn't long after that service that Jerry started getting very tired and began to slow down. He had gotten an infection and had to be hospitalized for twenty days. After he was dismissed from the hospital it was decided he should go to a rehabilitation facility.

He was extremely weak and couldn't care for himself, and I had returned to work. So he went into the facility on Wednesday and on Monday he became unresponsive and was taken back to the hospital. He went home to be with his Lord on Tuesday. Had God failed Jerry in the end? No! His last days were his best days. We had witnessed many miracles during our ministry but you might say the culmination of Jerry's ministry came two days after Jerry departed this life, I received a call from his sister, and she informed me that the young girl he had prayed for had conceived and expecting a baby. A miracle baby. The baby was born in October, close to Jerry's birthday. I was so thrilled, I put the phone down and thought, 'Oh I've got to tell Jerry!' But of course he knows.

I didn't need to tell him anything.

He was able to end his life doing what he loved—preaching the gospel, and fully knowing the miracle working God, he encouraged that young couple to believe the same miracle working God for a child that they desperately wanted to have.

I believe Jerry knew he had completed his work here on earth and gave up the struggle to stay, and just peaceably, very quietly fell into the open arms of Jesus.

When he was in the hospital for the last time and they said he was dying, I didn't believe them. He had been at death's door three times before and pulled through, so I thought he would this time also. But when they took him off the respirator, it hit home. He was departing this earth for his heavenly home. This new journey was something he had planned to do all of his born-again life.

God has done His part. When Jesus went to the cross, he had already been beaten with a whip and the word says, *"by His stripes we are healed."* All of our sickness and disease was taken care of before he went to the cross! What an amazing Jesus! When He was going through that time of terrible suffering '*we were on his mind.*'

I leaned down and whispered in Jerry's ear that it was alright if he wanted to go home and be with the Lord. I did not want to be selfish, but I was silently screaming on the inside for him to please stay here. He had been through so much, so I really could not blame him for wanting to go home to be with the Lord. He had three very serious infections that had attacked his body and his immune system had been so compromised from all the Chemo no fight was left. In addition he was in tremendous pain.

I watched as his breathing became more shallow. The nurse came into the room which was full of family, and she told us to give him lots of hugs and kisses, that his pulse was down to thirty, and that these were his final moments. We loved on him as much as we could. I saw him take his last breath. He beautifully and peacefully left his body to go be present with the Lord.

The game had ended, the cancer was gone, Satan lost, and we won, but the days ahead were a blur. We had to make the funeral arrangements. My role of cheerleader was over, and I am now on a different journey. A new path. I traveled down a very confusing path for several months after Jerry's passing. Jerry and I were together twenty-four years, and many of those years, we were together 24/7. I was no longer a wife, a pastor's wife, a caregiver, a cheerleader, or roles I had been before.

Now I was alone and wondering where I fit in, wondering what I could have done differently. And, of course, playing the blame game if only I had been a better wife, showed more compassion, had more faith, quit my job, stayed with him, etc. I was pondering many questions that naturally come with the loss of a loved one.

Not just my own, but other people's questions, too. Some of the family members could not understand why Jerry departed at such a young age, especially when he was a strong man of faith. He stood in faith, he believed he received when he asked. So why is he in heaven now?

I'm sure the same questions are in other people's minds, and I would like to address those a little more. How does dying speak victory?

There are some things we can't answer, but this I know . . . GOD wants us to live strong and live long. Yes, the scripture says all men will die, but there is not a specific date for that departure in God's mind, Sometimes our choices about the food we eat, and the treatment of our bodies (the Temple of the Holy Ghost) take years off of our lives.

First let me say that I am so thankful when Jesus saw that he was coming prematurely, He opened His arms and welcomed him home.

Do not picture Jerry sitting on a cloud, playing a harp. No, he is working together with the Father, His Son, Jesus, the Holy Spirit and all the host of heaven. Another thing I know is that God works everything together for good for those who love Him. My husband definitely loved God.

Romans 8:28 *'And we know that all things work together for good to them that love God, to them who are thee called according to his purpose.'*

Jerry is still a part of those things that are working for our good.

He was busy about the Father's business on earth. He is busy about the Father's business in heaven. He is happy, whole, healed, and perfect. I can visualize him talking to people, comparing life experiences, that is if he will allow them to talk!

You had to know him. We would go to have lunch with our former Pastors at the 'Fiesta Grande' restaurant in Beardstown, Illinois, and what a wonderful experience listening to our husbands discuss the Bible!

Pastor Jerry and Pastor Gary would constantly go back and forth discussing enlightenment they would receive about the word of God while Pastor Pam (Pastor Gary's wife) and I would hardly get a word in edgewise. We were blessed to sit there in pride as we listened to our husbands.

Jerry is now being enlightened about the word of God now that he's home in heaven. When Jerry left us, there was a great shift in the heavenlies in 2009. Along with my husband's departure, more great men of God went home to be with the Lord, leaving empty places in the body of Christ—Billy Joe Daugherty, Oral Roberts among others.

They're not retired. They're alive! But who will receive their mantles on earth?

The body of Christ is like a big glove with many fingers working together to make a glorious church. There are the apostles, prophets, pastors, teachers and evangelists, known as the five-fold ministry.

In the church are great connections; ministers which will work together with each other fulfilling God's purpose—they are the glue.

There is a great preparation going on in heaven right now for the return of the Lord to this earth, and Jerry is a part of the biggest move God is going to make since Jesus departed earth—**His return**.

Who wouldn't love that role?

Losing anyone we love is never easy. If you have a loved one that has departed this earth, your job may be tougher now because a great physical distance is now between you and them. But be sure, someday soon heaven and earth will only be separated by your thoughts and not by miles.

After we have a chance to get our wits about us, we can now be happy and excited for them because we know they have inherited their *higher calling* in the Kingdom of God. The earthly calling is only a practice run for what's to come! Heaven is the goal, and he made it! We often forget heaven and earth are so closely connected together. We that are left on earth are diplomats, in close connection with those that have departed, with the same goal, which is fulfilling the *purpose of God*. Jerry fulfilled his purpose on earth. He's now fulfilling it in heaven.

> *I Corinthians 5:1 For we know that if the earthly tent which is our house is torn down, we have a building from God, a house not made with hands, eternal in the heavens.*

I pray this book, written from my heart, has been a blessing and encouragement to you, and may God bless you on your road to recovery. Remember, sometimes it does not come as fast as you would like. Sometimes you might have to be in recovery for awhile during your restoration period. Be sure to believe beyond what you feel. Be sure to believe beyond what you might be seeing your loved one go through. Faith sees beyond the present circumstance. Believe what the *Word of God* says about your situation!

One final scripture that has been a verse that has given me major strength . . . found in the Amplified Bible:

Jeremiah 29:11., For I know the thoughts and plans that I have for you, says the Lord, thoughts and plans for welfare and peace and not for evil, to give you hope in your final outcome.

In King James it reads:

Jeremiah 29:11 . . .

For I know the thoughts that I think toward you, saith the Lord, thoughts of peace, and not of evil, to give you an expected end.

Its not over we are a constant reminder in the eyes of the Lord and He is a constant reminder in our eyes that we are in a covenant relationship with each other. (We have each others back side.)

A *LOVE* relationship that shall never end

REJOICE!

Prayer for Healing!

Father, I thank you for sending Your Word to heal me. You are, the Word Jesus, You became flesh and dwelt among us. You bore my grief's (pains) and carried my sorrows (sickness). You were pierced through for my transgressions and crucified for my iniquities, the chastisement for my well being fell upon you and by your stripes I am healed. I Peter 2:24

Father, I thank you that Christ has redeemed me from the curse of the law, being made a curse for me. Deut 28:61 says _____ (name your sickness) is a curse of the law. Gal 3:13 says, "Christ has redeemed me from the curse of the law, therefore I am redeemed from _____.

Father, I thank you I'm your workmanship, created in your image for your good works which you prepared before hand that I should walk in them!

I John 5:14-15 And this is the confidence that we have in him, that, if we ask anything according to his will, he heareth us; And if we know that he hear us, whatsoever we ask, we know that we have the petitions that we desired of him.

It is **always** God's will to heal-we should never pray, "Father, <u>if it is your will, heal me</u>." God is love and always wants good things for his children!

Believe it, receive it and then Praise God for It!

Prayer for Salvation and Baptism in the Holy Spirit

Heavenly Father I come to You in the Name of Jesus. Acts 2:21 says, "Whosoever shall call upon the name of the Lord shall be saved" I am calling on You and asking you to come into my heart and be Lord over my life. Romans 10:9-10 says, "If thou shalt confess with thy mouth the Lord Jesus and shalt believe in thine heart that God raised him from the dead thou shalt be saved. I do that now, I confess that Jesus is Lord, and I believe in my heart that God raised Him from the dead. I am now born again! I am a Christian—a child of the Almighty God! I am saved!

You also said in Your Word, "If ye then, being evil, know how to give good gifts unto your children: HOW MUCH MORE shall your Heavenly Father give the Holy Spirit to them that ask him?" (Luke 11:13) I'm asking You to fill me with the Holy Spirit. Holy Spirit, rise up within me as I praise God. I fully expect to speak with other tongues as You give me the utterance (Acts 2:4) in Jesus Name. Amen!

Begin to praise God for filling you with the Holy Spirit. Speak those words and syllables you receive—not your own language, but the language the Holy Spirit gives you. God will not force you to speak. Don't be concerned with how it sounds. It is a heavenly language! You are a born again, Spirit Filled Believer—Your life will never be the same! Find a good church to attend—one that speaks the Word with Boldness and obeys it.

References:

* Healing Scriptures . . . . .Author Kenneth E. Hagin, Sr.
* Healed of Cancer . . . . .Author Dodie Osteen
* A Praying Wife . . . . .Author Stormie O'Martian
* A Place Called Heaven . . . Author Dr. Gary Wood

* Dr. Kim Wyatt MD-Beardstown Rural Health Clinic, Beardstown, Il

* Dr. Delva-Deauna-Oncologist, Kansas University Medical Center, Kansas City, Ks.

Only the Spirit knows when to leave a broken body behind!
Quote: The Movie "The Healer"

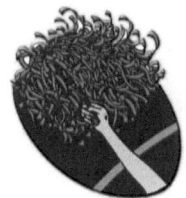

Cheerleader Faith
Team Spirit for the Cancer Patient
What to do When Trouble Comes

PHOTO GALLERY

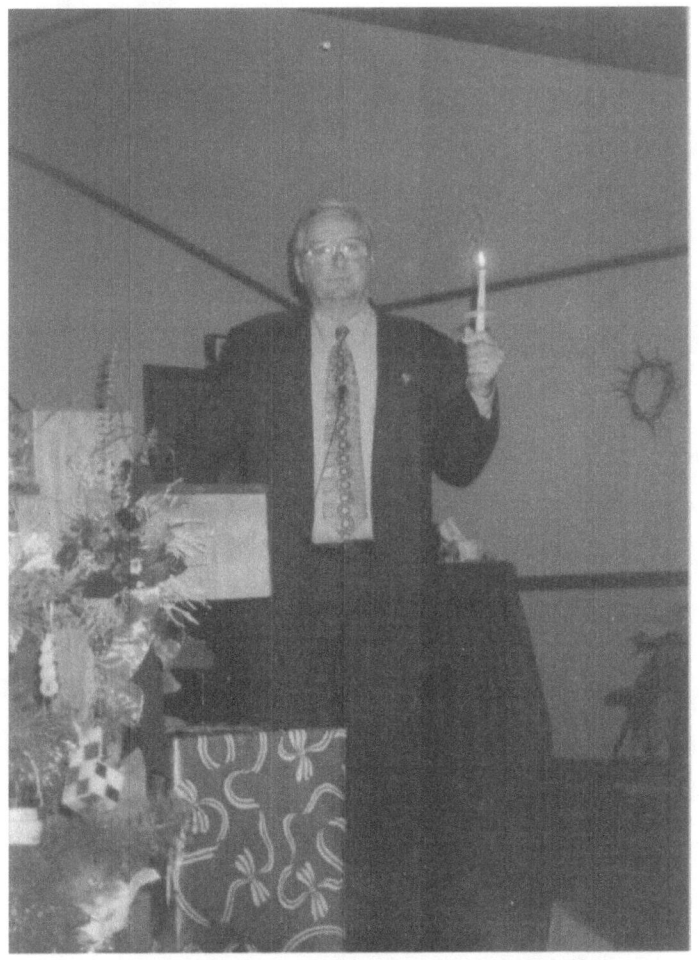

Candle Light Service–New Years Eve

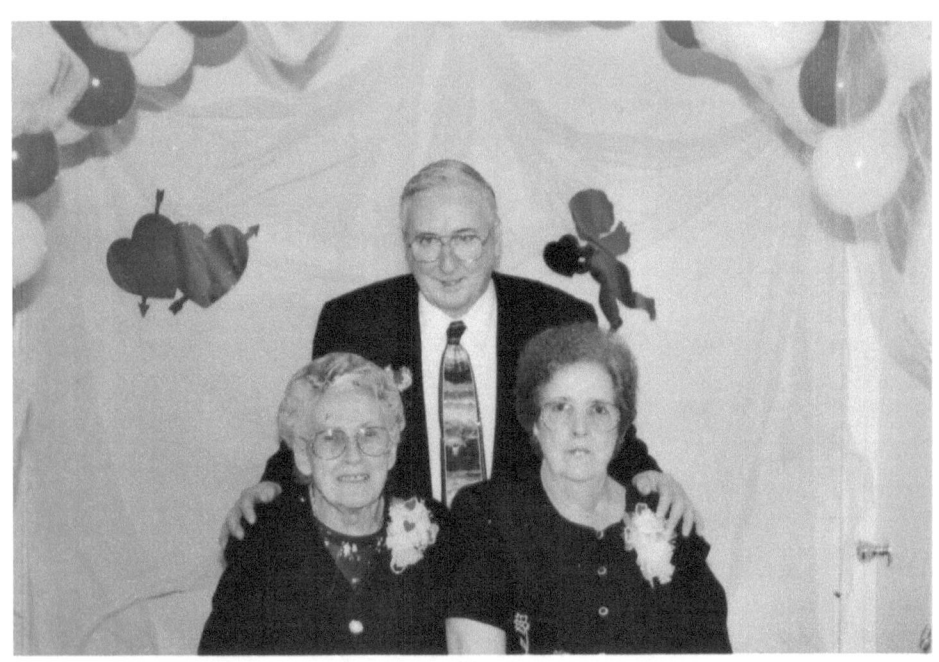

Pastor Jerry with his mother Opal and sister Wilma

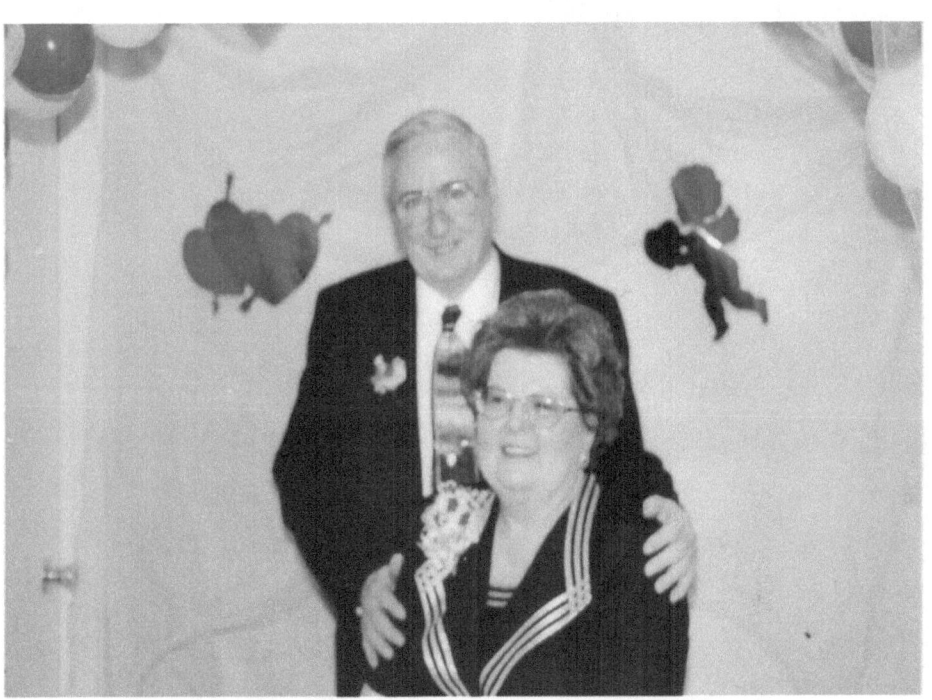

Sweetheart Banquet–Lighthouse Church–Jerry and Marge

CHEERLEADER FAITH

Team Spirit for the Cancer Patient
What To Do When Trouble Comes!

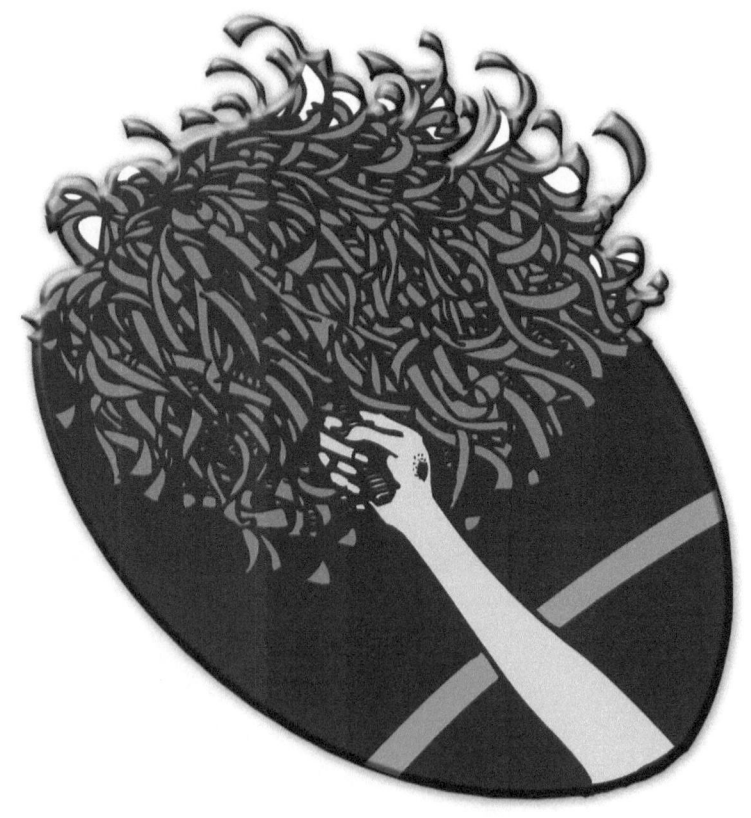

MARGE HOUCHINS